What Does ADHD Look Like?

Real Life Stories of Students
Told by the Educator
Who Worked with Them

by
Dr. Linda Salinas, Ed.D.

This book is a work of nonfiction. Names have been changed to protect privacy.

ISBN: 9781092417181

What Does ADHD Look Like?

Real Life Stories of Students
Told by the Educator
Who Worked with Them

Forward

I began my teaching career in elementary school. Well, maybe it wasn't the beginning of my *career*, but my friends and I played 'school' every day during recess when we were very young. We played 'school' in the summer, rotating between being the teacher and being the student.

Naturally, I majored in education when I attended college. Deciding on working with older students, I majored in secondary education. My first teaching job right out of college was in the Aldine Independent School District. I did student teaching at MacArthur High School in the fall, so the administrators had the chance to see my teaching before hiring me. I was hired at mid-term which is usually a difficult time to find a teaching job. I started off teaching several classes of government, a one semester course. In addition, I was hired to teach a course called Power, Personality, and Politics. Sounds interesting, doesn't it? I certainly thought so; I was very interested in politics. I didn't really learn until I was told I had the position, that the course had no curriculum. It was supposed to be about famous people throughout history who were leaders in government around the world. There was no textbook--- nothing. The teacher was supposed to design the course and teach it----and, by the way, class started in a week.

I was so excited about getting a high school position that I didn't care! In the first few days, I told my students that they would have the opportunity to actual design the course. They could select the personalities that they wanted to study and we would plan the course together. When would high school students ever actually have the opportunity to do that? They were excited! We divided into teams who did research and then prepared presentations. Some teams had films, some had costumes, and some brought in artifacts. My students did a better job planning the curriculum for this new one-of-a-kind course than I could have ever done. I was so proud.

After that first year and after I was feeling good about teaching government, I was visited by the principal of the school. He walked up to my classroom at the end of the hall on the second floor. That's scary! Did I do something wrong? I rarely saw the principal!

IIc was so kind but appeared to be very apologetic. He started off by saying, "You know, sometimes things change and we have to make adjustments." *What? Are you telling me I am going to lose my job? What else could it be?* These things went through my head in the two seconds after he made his first sentence.

"Our numbers change and sometimes we have to make adjustments so that all the classes are covered. We need you to teach English next year instead of government." *Whew!* I must have looked totally relieved!

"That's OK," I said with such a great sense of relief. "English is another one of my teaching fields (of course he already knew that) and I did my student teaching in English here with Carrie Durley."

"I know that," he said. "I just didn't want to disappoint you if you had your heart on teaching government."

Little did he know, I'd teach basket weaving just to have a high school teaching job.

When fall rolled around, I taught a full schedule of English classes and I loved every minute. I had started working on my master's degree in special education with certification to become an educational diagnostician.

An opening came up the following year teaching learning disabled students in the resource room. I had 29 boys and one girl. Since there were 6 class periods in the day, I only had around five students per period. In addition, I had a teaching assistant. *How good is this?* In some ways I missed teaching in the regular classroom, but this position enabled me to work with students very closely, and I could help them be successful. Most of my teaching was in the math area. I loved it. I loved my students. Is that where my love of tutoring began?

I completed my master's degree. The following year, and after only two and one-half years teaching, I was offered the position as educational diagnostician. It was a higher paying job but meant that I would be moving from the high school to two middle schools in the school district. It meant leaving all the friends I had made at the high school; it meant leaving the resource students that I helped and might possible have again the following year. I would miss them.

The years I worked as a diagnostician set the stage for a private testing practice that I engaged in when I moved to Dallas in 1978 after six years of experience in the Aldine district. The district served me so well, and I have so much to thank them for. They gave me the opportunity to get experience as a high school regular teacher, a high school resource teacher, and an educational diagnostician.

A personal relationship instigated the move from Houston to Dallas. I was offered yet another job in Aldine to be the lead diagnostician in their new high school. It would have been a large promotion. I was told that the reason I was being offered the job when I had less experience than most of their other diagnosticians (I think there were 16 diagnosticians in the district at that time.) was that I did twice the amount of work than most of the others. I thanked them for their vote of confidence and for the compliment. However, I had to tell the personnel director and special education director that I had already made plans to move to Dallas. If I were remaining in Aldine, I would have accepted the position instantly! But–I wasn't. I was moving to Dallas without a position at all! Was I crazy?

As luck would have it, I was able to secure a position as educational diagnostician for the Highland Park Independent School District in the Dallas area. I soon found out that HPISD was one of the best school districts in the nation. In fact, it was ranked twelfth in the nation around that time.

HPISD was a small district and a huge change from the very large district I had worked in before. I would be the second diagnostician. With only two diagnosticians, each of us would be responsible for three schools. My partner had once been a kindergarten teacher, so she preferred working with younger children. With my experience, I took the middle school, high school, and students who needed to be tested at the elementary school that she couldn't get to. My office was in one of the elementary schools. What was so great was getting experience at all levels and being in all of the schools. I met so many fantastic educators!

After several years of working as an educational diagnostician, a position opened for the newly developed job as teacher appraiser. The state of Texas required all teachers be evaluated every year.There were two teacher appraisers— myself and one other person. I loved every minute of that job. How lucky I was to get to go into classrooms all day long and observe wonderful teachers doing a great job of teaching. *Every day!* Then, I met with each teacher and had the privilege of complimenting them on what a great job he or she had done. Sometimes I had constructive ideas for improvement, and the teachers seemed to enjoy that, also.

After a couple of years as teacher appraiser, a position opened for assistant principal at the high school where my office was located. I had completed my doctorate by this time, and I majored in educational administration with certification as a superintendent. That assistant principal job would be just perfect for me, I thought.

I told those who interviewed me that I thought it was the hardest job in the district based on the fact that the hours were very long—assistants were expected to be at games and events almost every evening until late. In addition, assistants were the ones who administered discipline. That is never an easy job. "Knowing that this job is one of the hardest in the district, I still want it." I told the selection committee.

The interesting thing about the job was that it was going to be a half time job. I would be a teacher appraiser for one half of the time and would be assistant principal with two other assistants for one half of the time. Do you know that two half time jobs *does not* equal one full time job? It comes more closely to equaling 1.25 of a job. One job tends to carry over into the next job and one person ends up doing both for the majority of the time.

The following year turned out to be fulltime assistant principal. I loved the job, and I loved working with students, teachers, and parents. I learned so much in that position. I learned that all students want to do well, and they want to do the right thing. Sometimes, peer pressure and lack of maturity push them into situations they don't like being in but they don't know how to get out of them.

When our principal left unexpectedly over the summer, I was tagged to be the interim high school principal. "Just keep the place running," the superintendent said to me. "Don't do anything new and don't change anything. We will hire a principal with previous high school principal experience to take over at the end of the year."

I knew that the superintendent wanted a principal with lots of experience running a high school from another district and even from another state. At the end of the year, an experienced principal from a northern state was brought in to assume the position as principal.

When asked if I would move to central office to take a position there, I voiced that I really wanted more principal experience before a central office position. He graciously allowed me to become the 7-8 middle school principal. I already knew the teachers from being the teacher appraiser there, and they were comfortable with me. Besides, in another year, we were going to get to move into the brand-new school---the first new school in the district in almost 80 years! What fun!

Several professionals at central office were leaving, so after only two years of working as the middle school principal, I was tapped to be the director of instruction at central office. This time I had no choice in the decision—I was going.

In many ways, I hated to leave the middle school. I loved the students—the teachers—the parents—and all of the support staff workers. In another way, I realized that I could still be connected but could have a more important role in decision making at the central level for the entire district.

In my new position, I was asked to supervise and facilitate nurses, counselors, principals, and coaches. I was responsible for curriculum guide reviews and development, new teacher orientation, and basically everything no one else wanted to do. Really! It was a difficult year. I had so many responsibilities I had to write them on a flip chart in my office, so I could review them daily.

After two years, an opening came up for director of personnel. I had once owned a personnel agency with my sister, so I thought it would be the perfect fit. I was given the position and loved every minute of it. Actually, every job I ever had since being hired as a teacher in 1973 was perfect in my eyes. I loved each and every position.

I retired from the position of director of personnel after a tenure of 7 years. I retired young, age 52, after a total of 9 different positions over 29 years. How blessed I was to have experienced such a variety of positions in my career. I learned valuable lessons from each and every one.

I continue to be involved in education. Today, I tutor students every day of the week, test students for learning disabilities and other learning problems, screen students for the Texas A&M Dental School (for the past 15 years), and prepare students to take the SAT and ACT. I learn more from my students then they learn from me.

I reviewed my various career changes to say that I am looking at ADHD through the eyes of many different positions in the educational field: teacher, special educational teacher, diagnostician, assistant principal, principal, director of instruction, director of personnel, and tutor.

That brings me to why I wanted to write this book on ADHD difficulties. I think it can be very helpful to parents and teachers. What Does ADHD Look Like? Hopefully, these stories will give *you* insight and answers to that question.

What Does ADHD Look Like?
Real Life Stories of Students
Told by the Educator
Who Worked with Them

Chapter One
A Variety of Experiences in Education

I'm not a medical doctor. I can't prescribe medication for any condition. I'm an educator who cares about finding out why any student is having difficulty in school. Every student really wants to do well, even if he pretends that it doesn't matter. I want to help those students. I want them to have good, positive experiences in their school or learning environment. I've had quite a bit of training, but no training in the world takes the place of actual experience working one-to-one with students.

I look at students from the eyes of all of the positions I have held: teacher, special education teacher, educational diagnostician, teacher appraiser, high school assistant principal, interim high school principal, middle school principal, director of instruction, director of personnel, and tutor.

As a teacher, I looked at students as they sat in my class. I noticed if they were attentive and engaged or inattentive and disengaged. I noticed if they turned in homework and assignments, or if they struggled to do so. I looked at how they did on quizzes and exams. I looked at their activity level in class or if they were lethargic. I made mental notes.

As special education teacher (special education resource teacher), I worked with students on a one-to-one basis. I saw their attention level even in a one-to-one situation. It was obvious when students were hyperactive and couldn't stay still for even a few minutes. It was obvious when a student learned a concept one day and then forgot it for the next day. I made mental notes.

As an educational diagnostician, I tested hundreds of students in the public-school system but also tested many students in a private setting. Even when students were trying to do well, students with ADHD struggled to stay focused and on task. The testing showed gaps in learning even when the intelligence level was very high. Students with an ADHD profile demonstrated difficulties in the test setting. The picture became clear. I made mental notes.

When I became a teacher appraiser, I spent the majority of every day sitting in regular classrooms observing not only the teacher, but also the students. I could see how the students were reacting to the lecture or the teaching activity. I could pick out the students who were inattentive or hyperactive. I could see how these students fared in various classrooms and why they lost much of the instruction on a daily basis. I made mental notes.

I saw an entirely different perspective when I became an assistant principal at the high school. I saw more behavioral problems that probably had their roots in ADHD difficulties. As an assistant principal, parents frequently entered the picture. I witnessed the interaction between student and parent. I made mental notes.

As interim principal of the high school, the seriousness of behavioral issues and ADHD difficulties was heightened. Parents were finely tuned into grade point averages for college admission. Every issue was important. I made mental notes.

As principal of the middle school, I noticed a huge difference in level of importance as perceived by the parents. They were interested in grades but not at the level that I saw at the high school. Parents were more concerned if behavior was an issue, but grade point average wasn't as important. I made mental notes.

Once I moved into central administration positions, I was not in direct contact with students, as I had been for almost twenty years. Now, my perspective was based on discussions with principals and teachers. I made mental notes.

Although I didn't work directly with students during the day while I worked at central office, I tutored students from several cities in the metroplex on almost a daily basis. I saw the homework assignments, the test expectations, and the workload administered in both public schools as well as private schools. I continued with a private practice conducting individual psychoeducational evaluations, and local pediatric clinics referred students to me for testing. I made mental notes on my experiences.

My experience with psychoeducational evaluations has led me to work with Dr. Peter Ray, M.D., a specialist in ADHD difficulties. He has several excellent handouts that explain the various types of medications and potential side effects. He puts his heart and his soul into finding just the right medication to do what is necessary to get the student on track to success. I have referred many students to him, and I see very positive results.

Dr. Peter Ray, M.D. works diligently to get the right medication for each student. He is the only medical doctor in my forty plus years of experience who called me at home in the evening to discuss students that I referred to him. He had many questions to ask me concerning the student's ability to focus when we were tutoring or the student's demeanor or overall personality. He really cares about the success of the student. He once told me, "Success stories are what keeps me going. That's why I do what I do."

In his handout to parents, he lists the potential side effects of stimulant medications including: decreased appetite, insomnia, excessive moodiness and irritability, headache, stomachache, and motor tics. The potential side effects of tricyclic antidepressants include drowsiness initially, dry mouth, headache, stomachache, constipation, skin rash, irritability or depression, or disturbance of heart rhythm (only high doses). Therefore, if a parent notices any of these side effects, let the doctor know in case he wants to decrease the dosage or choose another medication.

Over the past forty-seven years, my life has been consumed with working with parents, teachers, administrators, psychologists, psychiatrists, and medical doctors to help students. More importantly, for the past forty-seven years, I have worked with students to help *them*.

I'd love to hear your stories. My email is dr.lindasalinas@vcrizon.net

Chapter Two
Collection of ADHD Stories

For many years, I told parents and students stories of other students who had been diagnosed with ADHD and how the diagnosis actually changed their lives for the better. I said a million times, "I need to write a book! There are so many stories that I have told over the years, and the stories keep coming."

I finally found the time to write those stories down. These are stories that I have been personally involved in. They are stories of my own students, parents of my students, or family members or friends. Some of the names are real, some of the names have been changed to protect their privacy, and many of the names are different because I can't remember the actual name. **This is a way to put a real face on what ADHD looks like.** I hope this helps parents understand that sometimes the child they have who doesn't try—or is lazy—or doesn't study—is really suffering from ADHD.

There is another way to solve the problem.

What is important to also understand is that parents do not see their child the same way that teachers see him. Parents will not understand, unless they are able to become invisible and can sit in the classroom with their child. Some parents see a little of what their students experience, if they work with them on homework in the evening. It is still different in the actual classroom. When I hear parents say that their child is lazy, doesn't seem to care, doesn't try to study, never turns in homework, and the other usual comments, I always suspect ADHD.

Another interesting point is that very frequently, one or both parents have a difficulty with ADHD but don't even realize it. Adults who have difficulty with time and organization may have ADHD difficulties. If adults talk excessively, it is a sign. If adults always lose things, or forget where they put them, it is sign. Generally, people who are around ADHD adults just learn to cope with the inconveniences.

If this book can help parents understand that their child's difficulty may actually be a form of ADHD and ADHD can be helped, then it has been successful.

Chapter Three
Is it ADD or ADHD? I'm confused.

Sometimes parents tell me that their child is ADD but not ADHD because he is not hyperactive. In reality, the two terms are the same. ADD is the older term. Like most things, terms change over time. The same holds true for ADD. Over time, it changed from ADD (Attention Deficit Disorder) to ADHD (Attention Deficit-Hyperactivity Disorder). It was 1994 when the new term was put into place. ADD still continues as the generic term. But now, a diagnosis can be more specific. In the Diagnostic and Statistical Manual of Mental Disorders code book (DSM), ADHD is listed three ways: ADIID-Inattentive; ADHD-Hyperactive; and ADHD-Combined Type. The following information is taken directly from the DSM-IV-TR quick reference guide.

ADHD-Predominately Inattentive

This diagnosis is given if a child has six or more symptoms of inattention for at least six consecutive months to a degree that is maladaptive and inconsistent with developmental level. The symptoms are:

1) often fails to give close attention in tasks or play activities
2) often has difficulty sustaining attention in tasks or play activities
3) often does not seem to listen when spoken to directly
4) often does not follow through on instructions and fails to finish schoolwork, chores, or duties in the workplace (not due to oppositional behavior or failure to understand instruction)
5) often has difficulty organizing tasks and activities
6) often avoids, dislikes, or is reluctant to engage in asks that require sustained mental effort (such as schoolwork or homework)

7)   often loses things necessary for tasks or activities (e.g, toys, school assignments, pencils, books, or tools)
8)   is often easily distracted by extraneous stimuli
9)   is often forgetful in daily activities

ADHD-Predominately Hyperactive

This diagnosis is given if a child has six or more symptoms of hyperactivity-impulsivity for at least six consecutive months to a degree that is maladaptive and inconsistent with developmental level. The symptoms are:

Hyperactivity:

1)   often fidgets with hands or feet or squirms in seat
2)   often leaves seat in classroom or
in   other situations in which remaining seated is expected

3) often runs around or climbs excessively in situations in which it is inappropriate (in adolescents and adults may be limited to subjective feelings of restlessness)

4) often has difficulty playing or engaging in leisure activities quietly

5) is often "on the go" or often acts if "driven by a motor"

6) often talks excessively

Impulsivity:

7) often blurts out answers before questions have been completed

8) often has difficulty awaiting turn

9) often interrupts or intrudes on others (e.g., butts into conversations or games)

For diagnosis, the following things must be met:

a) Either six or more symptoms of inattention or hyperactivity-impulsivity exists.

b)   Some hyperactive-impulsive or inattentive symptoms that caused impairment were present before age 7 years.

c)   Some impairment from the symptoms is present in two or more settings (at school or work, and at home).

d)   There must be clear evidence of clinically significant impairment

in   social, academic, or occupational functioning.

e)   The symptoms do not occur exclusively   during the course of a Pervasive   Developmental Disorder, Schizophrenia,   or other Psychotic Disorder and are not better accounted for by another mental disorder (e.g., Mood Disorder, Anxicty Disorder, Dissociative Disorder, or a Personality Disorder).

Chapter Four
Seven Specific Kinds of ADHD

Most people think there are only two different kinds of ADHD difficulties: inattentive or hyperactive. In reality, there are many different kinds of ADHD and they can overlap. They are often not clear cut. Dr. Daniel Amen, M.D. explains the seven different kinds of ADHD in his book titled <u>Healing ADD: The Breakthrough Program that Allows You to See and Heal the 7 Types of ADD.</u> I highly recommend this book for a more thorough understanding of the science behind ADHD.

For organizational purposes, I will organize stories of my experiences with students under the seven main types presented in Dr. Amen's book.

Many parents over the years have told me that they know their child isn't ADHD, because he can sit and work on video games for long periods of time. Children with ADHD *can* sit for long periods of time, if they are interested in the task. It is regular, routine, or boring tasks that the student cannot do. Hopefully, reading about these *real* students with *real* ADHD difficulties will help parents understand more about what ADHD actually looks like.

Classic ADD (ADHD)

This category is what people always think about when thinking about ADHD, and it is the easiest one to diagnose. Students with Classic ADD are inattentive and highly distractible. They are disorganized and find difficulty in keeping anything organized or neat. Their backpacks are filled with extra papers that should be discarded. Their notebooks are crammed full of papers, many of which are falling out of the notebook. There is no organization to any notebook. Their desks or work areas at home are stacked high with miscellaneous books and papers and hobbies. Drawers and closets are packed and disorganized. Basically, their "stuff" is everywhere. Parents will typically try to organize their child. The mother may organize his notebook, organize his backpack, and organize his desk or work area. It stays organized as long as the parent is doing it for the child. Once the parent quits, the backpack, notebook, and work area become cluttered the way it was before. In this category, there is also some level of hyperactivity and restlessness. These students have difficulty with time and are frequently late or hurried. They are late in turning in projects and homework, because they don't realize how much time is needed to complete the task. They will tell you that they are "on their way" when they are an hour away from the time that they will even be leaving the house.

The Classic ADHD child is usually easily identified as a young child. Babies who are colicky and are very active fit this category. They are difficult to soothe and are sometimes hard to hold. Because they are hyperactive and conflict-driven, they get identified early. They tend to be noisy and demanding.

Chad

Chad was a young child who drove all the teachers crazy. He was in constant motion and got up out of his desk as often as he possibly could. There were reports that he actually fell out of his desk because of his high level of movement. Walking down the hallway, he seemed to bounce off the sides of the hallway like a pinball machine. His mother told us that children didn't like to play with her son, because he was so rough with them. He never got invited to go to anyone's house to play.

Finally, his mother took him to his pediatrician who prescribed medication for ADHD. Within a couple of weeks, everything changed significantly. The teachers noticed a huge difference and would actually ask the receptionist in the school office to call his mother if it were suspected that he forgot to take his medication. The teachers could tell just by watching him. After medication, Chad's mother reported that he now has friends who come over to play with him.

Carter

Carter was a student who always struggled with staying in his seat at school. Although the teachers tried to use behavior modification with Carter, it was never quite successful. They discussed their concerns with his parents, but his parents didn't know what to do, either. So, the teachers just tried to make it work and managed to get through the year. Since his activity continued the following year, his parents decided to look into supplements and medication for hyperactivity. First, they tried natural supplements, but they saw no improvement. Finally, they tried medication through their physician, and it appeared to be working to some extent. Just when the parents thought everything was going to be fine, Carter started acting out at home. He was openly defiant with his parents and talked back to them in a disrespectful way. Even when his parents punished him, he'd fight back. He'd scream and yell and tell them how much he hated them. They remained calm, telling him that they loved him even if he didn't love them, but nothing got better. Sometimes Carter would turn on himself, saying that he was stupid and he couldn't do anything right. His parents didn't know what to do. Consulting their physician, the parents agreed to a stronger ADHD medication that would address his anger more effectively. That seemed to work. Carter's activity level became more normal, and he did not have outbursts of defiance and anger. Remember, your physician does not know what is going on, unless you tell him or her. The physician needs your input. Adjustments can be made but only with the right communication.

Johnny

Johnny was a very likable student. He had the type of personality that every teacher loved. He didn't cause any trouble, and he was never a disruption in class. Although he struggled with his grades, he *appeared* to be listening in class. His tutor noticed there were large gaps in his learning. She didn't understand how he was unable to work basic math problems, yet he was in far more advanced math classes. Although he managed to get his assignments in, he was totally disorganized in everything he did for school. His notes were in total disarray. They were scattered around on the tabletop. His notes were on different sheets of paper, and they never appeared again. It seemed that he lost every note he ever took. Even the notes for SAT and ACT were totally disorganized. He felt compelled to write things down but then never knew where anything was. The tutor started keeping his notes in her office so that he would at least have his notes to look at, before he took the test. The tutor could keep them together, but if he left with them, they would be gone forever.

The parents did everything they could to give John what he needed——a great plan for nutrition and eating healthy and all kinds of tutorial support. What they didn't realize was that Johnny had ADHD and needed medication to improve. They weren't fond of the idea of medication, so they tried a natural supplement first. The tutor saw no improvement. Even though Johnny appeared to be focused while she was instructing him, he just couldn't "think" through much of the instruction. He needed multiple lessons to learn some of the concepts. Where most students with ADHD couldn't continue working, Johnny almost couldn't stop working. He was driven. The teachers saw that in him, and they worked as hard as he did to ensure that he was successful. He was given extended time on the SAT because of his ADHD diagnosis which helped significantly, but medication was still needed. Finally, after several months, John was placed on ADHD medication which seemed to help significantly. He felt that he was picking up more information in class, and his homework did not take as long to finish. He was still scattered but seemed to be a little more organized with his notes and notebooks. There were still issues with Johnny that went beyond ADHD and his medical doctor recognized that. Johnny and his doctor are working through those issues.

Milly

Milly was a very sweet eighth grade student who had previously been identified as ADHD and was on medication. She had much difficulty with academic coursework and was provided with accommodations to be successful in her academic setting. I started tutoring her and noticed her hyperactivity and distractibility immediately. If a sight unusual noise was heard outside or in another room, she would be pulled in that direction. She always wanted to know what the noise was. "That's just the back door opening," I told her. Then she felt the need to discuss it. When I tried to explain something to her, she frequently

40

interrupted me several times so that I would have to start over on the explanation. That happened numerous times. Many times, I noticed that she didn't hear me at all. Keeping her focused on some days was nearly impossible. Since I suspected that her medication was not the right one, or the dosage needed to be adjusted, I discussed the issue with her parents. They agreed to ask her physician, but the situation did not improve. Sometimes, there doesn't seem to be anything that makes the situation better. Everyone on the student's team just tries to do the best that is possible. In Milly's case, I believe that she will be a successful member of society as an adult. She will find her niche and will do well. Her personality will help her become self-sufficient. Everyone who comes in contact with her likes her. But, she still struggles with focus. She needs to try a different medication. She will never be able to do well academically as long as her ADHD keeps her from focusing. She is in the process of working with her physician to get a different medication.

Inattentive ADHD

This category is for those students who are inattentive and easily distracted, but who are not hyperactive. By the time a student reaches the middle school years, he or she is usually an expert in hiding this diagnosis from his teacher. He can make eye contact and appear to be taking notes, but he is not hearing a word the teacher is saying. His mind is somewhere else. The teacher may not know he is not engaged, unless she calls on him for an answer to a question. Then, he will typically ask the teacher to repeat the question. Sometimes, students can just sit and daydream. They may seem spacey. They are often perfectly happy sitting around not doing anything. They appear to be quite laid back. These students have difficulty listening when someone else is talking. They also have a difficult time being organized in their work area. Time is also an issue, so homework tends to be late. These students tend to make careless mistakes. They complain about being bored or they appear unmotivated. These students may appear tired, sluggish or very slow moving.

Blake Taylor's book titled ADHD & Me explains ADHD-inattention this way: "When distraction---and therefore the inability to concentrate-----occurs, I feel as if my mind were a television with the channel changing uncontrollably."

Susan

Susan was a really sweet girl who came to me while in her sophomore year at the high school. Because she was so compliant and never caused her teachers any difficulty at all, her teachers assisted her as much as they could, but probably enabled her ADHD to continue unnoticed to her parents. She had difficulty turning in assignments on time. She would get points deducted from that assignment, but they would allow her to do extra credit when she could. There was no deadline on the extra credit, so time constraints didn't create difficulty for her. She had difficulty paying attention in class but was never disruptive or a disturbance in class. Her parents provided her with a tutor who taught her things she missed in class because of inattention. They did not realize that she actually had ADHD and could have learned so much better with the help of medication. When a student takes home a report card with all good grades, parents have no idea that there may be a real difficulty. Sometimes the difficulty doesn't start surfacing until the student goes to college. Then her SAT came back with a below average score. This was the first time that the parents noticed a difficulty. They thought it was just a fluke. How could she be such a good student, make good grades, yet score so low on the SAT? The teachers couldn't help her on her SAT score. She was on her own for that one and it showed.

Her parents decided to have her tested, now concerned that she might not get into the university that she wanted to enter.

The test results showed a significant level of inattention along with a processing speed difficulty. She didn't have time to finish the SAT and resolved to guessing on the last ten to twelve questions in each section. Her parents took her to a physician who prescribed ADHD medication. Within a month, Susan was doing much better. She said her learning experience was completely different. She could actually listen to the teacher and understand what was being said. She didn't get distracted as much and quit watching the clock for the class to be over. Even in doing her homework, she was able to focus on the task at hand and complete it in a normal amount of time. She felt she was "learning" for the first time.

Andrew

One of my favorite ADHD stories involves a student named Andrew. He was in the ninth grade when I first spoke to his mother. She knew he was very smart, but he was struggling with school and had difficulty making good grades. Although he was conscientious and worked hard, he continued to struggle in school with low test scores and lower grades than expected. Thinking another school setting would work better for Andrew, his mother moved him to a private school. It did not work for him. In addition to trying to adjust to a new environment, he didn't do well with the fact that he was required to attend every varsity football game and stand on the sideline, since he was an underclassman football player. He really needed that time to study and do homework. Although his mother said that she would move him back to his former school for the following year, I suggested she move him right away instead of waiting until the beginning of the next school year. Why make him suffer?

I started tutoring Andrew. In helping him with his math homework, I could see that he was struggling with attention and focus, and he was actually *suffering*. It was so obvious to me, working with him so closely, that he was trying very hard, but he lost his focus every few seconds. I felt that Andrew would benefit from ADHD medication. When I mentioned that to his mother, she voiced her concern. She replied that Andrew's father hated the thought of ADHD medication and felt that was more detrimental than good. They had a friend who was on medication, and they felt it was not a good thing. I loaned her my ADHD books, so she could read actual cases. We continued on. When Andrew came to work on homework once a week, I kept seeing that he was trying but was suffering from lack of focus.

Soon, he was into his sophomore year. Nothing had changed. His mother developed a program on an excel spreadsheet that basically required Andrew to work on schoolwork for two hours every evening in his room. Even if he had no homework or tests, he was required to work on schoolwork for two hours every evening. The theory sounds great, but I have been working with teenagers for forty years, and I felt that program would not work. It didn't. Soon, Andrew and his mother were having difficulties. She basically grounded him from using his vehicle, forcing him to catch a ride to school with his sister. That was humiliating to him. There were other grounding episodes. Then Andrew ran into a wall.

He came home one day and said he was going to quit school as soon as he could. He explained he was beating his head against the wall every day. He was totally discouraged. His self-image was low. He had always wanted to be a doctor and now that goal seemed to be impossible.

It wasn't until then that his mother called and asked what I recommended. I asked her to call a medical doctor whom I recommended. This doctor helped many of my students, and he was very sincere in finding the right medical solution.

It took a little time, but when Andrew and his mother finally got to talk to the doctor, medication was prescribed and Andrew was on his way. He told me that he felt a little funny the first week, because he actually felt a little aggressive. I asked him to give it time; his body was trying to adjust. Within one month, Andrew had adjusted to the medication, and he could tell a real difference. His grades started improving.

One day when he came for tutoring, he said, "You're going to love this."

"What?" I asked. "Tell me what I'm going to love."

"Well, I had a chemistry test, and I made a 94. It was the highest grade out of all of the classes."

On another occasion, he showed me a paper that he had done in class. The paper had a complete essay on the front and a very detailed drawing on the back.

"I did this in a 45-minute class!" he exclaimed. "I can't believe I did the whole thing in just one class period."

I was amazed also. He had to have been totally focused to have done all that work in one period.

One day when he came for math tutoring, we were working on some very difficult problems, and he was very focused on learning. Normally, students notice the clock, because they are ready to go after a full hour of work. I would be too! On this particular night, I allowed Andrew to continue working past the hour, since there was no student following him for tutoring. I wanted to see just how long it would take him to notice the time was up. We continued working for about 17 minutes before he figured it out.

"I'm so sorry!" he exclaimed. "We've gone over our time!"

"I know," I said. "I knew exactly what time it was, but I wanted to see how long you could stay focused. You could have never done that before medication."

Andrew told me one day, "You know, I think if I had had this medication my freshman year, I would have done pretty well."

"You absolutely would have." I said. "So, what does your father think about this now?" I knew that his father was not in favor of the medication.

"Oh, he's all over it now. He thinks he was the same way when he was a student growing up."

Later, Andrew told me of another interesting thing. Since he had the flu and missed several days of school, he was *way* behind in his classwork. His mother told him he could remain home, while the family attended church on Sunday, so that he could catch up. He told me that within two hours, he had completed all of his schoolwork. He then started cleaning out his closet and doing his own laundry.

I have heard other stories of productivity levels like this with students who have been on medication for ADHD. They are actually surprised at what they can accomplish.

Brian

Another one of my favorite stories involves a student who was in the tenth grade. His father called me and explained that his son was just not trying. He was not doing his work and was not studying. His father felt that he had also reached the end of the line as far as knowing what to do with Brian. I agreed to tutor him in math to try to get him caught up. My goal at that point was to get him to pass his algebra class.

When I started working with him, I could tell he was pretty smart, but he had big holes in his learning. There were gaps in his knowledge. Then it became obvious that he couldn't focus, either. No wonder there were gaps in his learning! He listened in class but was only getting instruction once in a while, not consistently. It would be very difficult to keep up in a math class, if you are not hearing everything the teacher is saying. I've explained it before like this: If you are listening to a lecture on the television, and the sound turns off every minute or so, you miss out on instruction. You are not hearing everything that you need to hear. It is the same thing with school. If a student cannot focus, he is missing out on some of the instruction. A really bright student can overcome that difficulty for at least a while, but it eventually catches up with him.

I asked the father to consider taking Brian to the same medical doctor to be checked out for ADHD medication. They did and in time, Brian could really notice a difference.

Brian even asked his father if he would order the math book that he would be using his junior year, so he could work through it over the summer. Did I hear that right? A sixteen-year-old boy wanting to get his math book, so he can study over the summer? I've been tutoring for over forty years and I have NEVER known that to happen.

Brian's father ordered the book and, sure enough, Brian started working in it. When he came for tutoring, he showed me page after page in a spiral notebook where he had worked problem after problem. He marked the ones that he wanted me to help him with. He was so proud of the fact that he had accomplished so much math on his own.
He referred to his life before ADHD medication as 'the time when I was not thinking.'

He even told one of his friends that he once only cared about watching videos and playing video games. "Now," he said, "I really want to get my work done." He was as surprised as anyone. He said, "I don't understand how that stuff works!"

Jed

I got a call from a parent who was totally distressed about her college son. He had failed almost all of his classes, and she didn't know what to do.

Jed was a bright student who managed to make it through high school in a small town in the Dallas suburbs. He played football and kept his grades up in order to continue playing. He did well enough to get accepted into Texas A&M which is not an easy task.

Jed finished his first semester with failing grades in most of his classes. His parents felt that he was partying too much and wasn't studying or completing his work. They felt that he was a typical high school student going off to college and not being able to be responsible. After a lecture on working hard and not partying, Jed replied that he *was* working hard, and he was not staying out late partying. They decided to allow him to stay there until the end of the year and then they would assess the situation.

Jed loved A&M so you know he wanted to do his best to stay there. But things didn't work out that way. He did just as poorly the second semester, so his parents moved him home where they could 'watch' him. They would make sure he was studying and not going out partying.

The school year began and he started attending classes through the community college. What they saw was interesting. He was studying every evening. He never went out partying. They were puzzled. He couldn't make his grades at the community college, either. Now, they were really worried!

Somehow, someone told them to visit with me. We talked and then decided to do testing. The testing was very clear. Test results indicated that Jed had a significant problem with not only focus and attention but also processing speed.

Jed's mother took him to their doctor and in a short time, he was on ADHD medication. It changed everything for him. He started making grades in the 90's at the community college. His friends knew he had difficulty before, so it was a shock to them also! They started asking him what he was doing to turn around his grades like he had done.

Jed came back to me later for tutoring in college algebra, and he said he didn't know that students learned that way until he took medication. He said, "I never knew that's how people learned."

He explained it this way to his friends: "If you can't see and then you get glasses, you go—wow! Now I can see. That is how it is with ADHD medication. You have difficulty learning and then—wow!—I can learn!"

James

James was a sixth-grade student when I started tutoring him in math. I could easily see from the beginning that he had trouble focusing. I would teach him a relatively easy concept and have him work a few problems on his own successfully, only to find that two minutes later, he couldn't do it. I would explain it again.

In a discussion with his mother, she decided to have him tested, again. The testing was clear—James had ADHD and processing issues. It was at the end of the year, so summer break was starting. When school started for his seventh-grade year, he started taking ADHD medication.

I had forgotten all about James's ADHD issue. I started working through his math sheet with him. Then he said, "Oh, I started on that stuff you told me about."

"What stuff?" I inquired.

"We went to the doctor and he gave me medicine so I can focus."

"Oh yes!! That's right! Is it helping?" I asked him.

"Can't you tell?" he asked me.

"Why yes! You are right! You have been focused this whole time! I just totally forgot. I can really tell the difference. Last year, I had to reteach because you were losing focus so often. What about at school? Can you tell it is helping you?"

"Yes," James said. "Before in every class, I used to just watch the clock and doodle. Now I can really listen to what the teacher is saying. I don't watch the clock anymore."

James started doing so well in school that he really didn't need tutoring any longer.

Jennifer

Jennifer was a high school senior whom I tutored for a couple of years. She had been diagnosed with ADHD when she was in elementary school and was still taking Ritalin for the disorder. Because she was going to play a sport in college, she was required to get a physical from her physician. During that physical, her doctor asked her, "Are you still taking Ritalin?" She responded that she was still taking Ritalin, since he originally prescribed it for her many years earlier. The doctor responded, "You are too old to be taking that now. I'm going to prescribe you another medication that will probably do a much better job."

Jennifer went on the other medication and noticed an improvement immediately. The next time I tutored her, she was excited to tell me how much it was helping her. "I used to get in from school and would procrastinate in doing my homework. I just couldn't get around to doing it. I let everything else get in the way. Now, I get home, grab a snack, and get right to my homework. I can get it done much faster, also. This is great. I wish I had been on this when I entered high school; I'm sure my grades would have been better!"

The lesson to be learned here is that sometimes a patient is placed on a medication, and if nothing is said to the doctor to indicate that the medication is not working, the prescription will be continued, sometimes indefinitely. Perhaps, like in this case, the student and the parents assumed the medication was working.

Sometimes parents don't notice anything wrong, since they are not at school with their son or daughter during the day, and often they don't get involved in their child's homework, either. They never question the medication. The student doesn't recognize a slow decline in his attention since it occurs over years. The student knows he is taking the medication prescribed by the doctor and doesn't question it.

One seminar I attended concerning ADHD presented a speaker who said it was important to monitor all ADHD medications closely because of the frequency that medications may need to be changed---either the type of medication or the dosage. Since the student's brain is still growing and changing, some medications may be better than others at certain times in the growth cycle.

Chances are, if Jennifer had changed to another medication even when she *entered* high school, she would have had a much easier time in studying and doing homework. One cannot predict the future, but it is interesting to consider it.

Collin

Collin came to me for SAT and ACT tutoring. Even though his scores were already very high, he wanted to shoot for that perfect score. He also came for help because he 'froze' on essays. He just couldn't get started. If he had an essay for homework, he couldn't do it. His thoughts would spin around and around and he could never get started. After we talked for a while, it seemed to me that he had that same mental block that can be common with students with some types of ADHD. I suggested he complete the Conner's Student Questionnaire and text me his answers. I entered his answers into the computer program that then generated his report. The results indicated that he had ADHD-Inattention. He wanted to have a parent conference to discuss his situation. I met his parents who indicated that ADHD was in their family and agreed with his self-diagnosis. Since he did not need any accommodations, other than medication, I suggested no psychoeducational testing. He ended up making a 36 (perfect score) on his ACT and will be a National Merit Scholar. He is anxious to see if medication will help him accomplish everything else he wants to do this summer—finish a book he wants to write; attend summer school; work on playing the French horn, piano, and guitar; and so many other things. His ambition shows that ADHD students can be highly accomplished, yet still have troubling difficulties.

Cindy

Cindy's mother came to me to discuss her daughter. Her daughter, Cindy, almost drowned when she was twenty-two months old.

Cindy was a very bright, precocious little girl who followed her older brother around all the time. She was so bright that her mother was told that she could go into the private school pre-kindergarten class earlier than normal. But when she was only 22 months old, she was found unresponsive in the family swimming pool.

It was the July 4th holiday. All of the kids were out in the pool enjoying the hot weather. Little Cindy walked out to the pool area, got too close to the edge of the pool, and fell in without anyone noticing. When it was noticed that she was missing, the family searched frantically. Cindy's mother moved a float in the pool to the horror of Cindy's little body underwater. Her mother pulled her little body out of the water and immediately began CPR. She had just been trained in CPR. Going into shock, Cindy's mom reasoned that her baby was dead. She walked into the house and continued making the salad for dinner. When Cindy's father caught up with them, he immediately called 911and the paramedics arrived quickly.

In the ambulance and at the hospital, emergency measures went into effect immediately. Cindy's parents were told that about one third of Cindy's brain was destroyed by the lack of oxygen and that they should consider placing her in a medical facility, because they would not be able to care for her. They said she would never walk, never talk, never be able to feed herself, and would basically be severely impaired for the rest of her life.

The parents would not accept that diagnosis. They took Cindy home, and they began working with her for hours every day. Her father worked in his job, and then he spent the next five hours working with Cindy. She could walk, could talk, and gradually overcame many of the obstacles that the doctors warned her parents about. But, everything took longer. When she wanted to ride her bicycle, it took eight hours for her to learn. Her parents gave her everything that she needed, so if she needed eight hours to learn to ride her bike, they were going to give that to her.

Since Cindy's recovery was exceptional in the doctors' eyes, they wanted to test her for everything. Finally, at the age of four, her parents decided that there would be no more testing. Cindy had been through enough!

The psychoeducational battery of tests given when she was older indicated an intelligence level in the deficient range. When Cindy's mother contacted universities concerning admission, she ran into a brick wall. When she explained about the near drowning and then answered their questions concerning Cindy's intelligence level, the university personnel always responded that their university did not have the services that Cindy needed.

When Cindy's mother met with me to discuss Cindy's future, I advised her to not offer any information about the drowning or the intelligence level. I explained that there is no accurate intelligence test that can measure a person's intelligence when an accident like the one Cindy had occurs. Besides, Cindy was making passing grades and she was a very good soccer player. In fact, she was a goalie and was one of the best players on the team.

When Cindy's mother asked if I could suggest anything further, I discussed the possibility of getting ADHD medication through Cindy's physician. "What if the medication does something in Cindy's brain that is positive?"

Cindy's mother went to the physician to ask his opinion. His first reaction was, "No, I don't think so."

"But, Doctor, after all that Cindy has gone through, shouldn't we try that? What if it really helps her?" Cindy's mother asked sincerely.

"Yes, you're right. Let's try ADHD medication," he agreed.

No one told the school personnel that Cindy was on a new medication. One of her teachers called her mother after about two weeks: "I don't know what you are doing differently with Cindy but her grade average is ten points higher than last grading period. She is focused in class and joins in on class discussions that she didn't do before. She's almost like a different student."

Then, one day, Cindy called home to talk to her mother: "Mom, don't ever take me off that medication. I made a B in my physics class. I've never done that well. I've never had a grade above 60."

When I saw Cindy to tutor her in algebra, I asked her if the medication helped her with her soccer. "I can't explain it, but I know I'm a better player now," she answered.

As it turned out, Cindy was accepted into a university and played for their soccer team. It was difficult academically, but she passed. Because she was injured in a game and was determined to have had a concussion, she had a scan of her brain. To her parents' surprise, Cindy's brain looked normal. It did not show the one-third damaged area that was seen when she had her drowning incident. It was like a miracle. Now, we know there is something called neuroplasticity. The brain can actually regenerate or redevelop in many areas. Research in that area is very interesting.

Cindy graduated from college and is currently working in her parents' real estate business. She is doing an excellent job and her skills for the business are increasing significantly.

It was just a guess that medication might do something for Cindy. In her case, it really did.

Lance

Lance was a very smart student who made it through high school relatively easily. His IQ was in the superior range. When he got to college, he encountered difficulty in his calculus class and ended up failing several tests. One of his friends suggested that Lance take on of his ADHD pills. Even though he knew that it was illegal to do so, Lance was desperate and tried it anyway. On the very next test, Lance made 94. He figured out that with

ADHD medication he could make in the 90's on tests, but if he didn't take the medication, he ran out of time and failed the tests. He finally confided in his mother what had been going on and she contacted me to see what we needed to do. I suggested that since Lance didn't seem to need any other accommodations such as extended time or a separate room to test in, I would have Lance and his mother complete a Conners' questionnaire. I put the numbers into the computer program which then produced several charts with results on ADHD scales. I included the results in a letter to Lance's physician asking for ADHD medication. The physician gave Lance Adderall, and he began taking it immediately. Lance couldn't believe the difference it makes in his attention and his study habits. His grade point average for his high school studies would have been significantly higher if he had been on medication while in high school. I'm just glad he figured it out during his freshman year in college! In talking with him later, he explained that every test that he took while on his medication was graded with an "A." Every test he took without medication was graded as a "B" or "C" and he usually ran out of time.

Lance told his mother that on the medication, he felt that he was awake for the 'second' time. In other words, he woke up in the morning, but on the medication, he felt that he was waking up again on a higher level. He could understand the information given in class. When he had to read on his own, he could focus and not have to read and reread.

Eve

After Lance figured out that medication was the key to passing calculus, he had a conversation with his sister who was two years younger and had just graduated from high school. Eve struggled in high school and barely finished her senior year. Her parents did not think she was mature enough to go off to college and decided to have her attend a community college and remain in the home setting another year. When Lance experienced an amazing transformation with ADHD medication, Eve asked her mother to consider it for her, also. Eve had always been told that she wasn't trying, that she was just lazy or wasn't applying herself. She was accused of not studying. Eve told me that she really was trying and she really *was* studying. We decided to do the same thing for Eve. She completed the questionnaires and the results were included in a letter to her physician. She was prescribed Adderall, also. I saw Eve at a function a couple of months later, and she looked great. She had lost weight because of the Adderall and she looked great, but it was what she told me in conversation that impressed me the most.

"I never knew that you could actually read a page in a book and remember what you read. I can listen to the teacher and remember what she said also. This is amazing!"

A couple of months after that, I ran into her grandfather who told me this.

"Eve was at our house the other day and she walked into the room with tears in her eyes. I thought, 'Oh, no—what has happened now?' I asked her what was wrong."

"Nothing's wrong. I just can't believe I can do this. I'm making "A's" in both of my college classes," she answered.

Both Lance and Eve were very intelligent students who were able to make it through high school, many times struggling, but who figured out after graduating that they were living with ADHD difficulties. Their mother, a school teacher, couldn't see that in them. Parents usually cannot.

Silvia

Silvia was a student who came to me for tutoring for the SAT and ACT. I knew that she got extended time to take the tests, so I inquired about medication. She explained that she had been on medication for just a short time. She was a junior and had gotten on medication during the second semester of her sophomore year.

"How did you know you needed to be on medication?" I asked.

"Well, I struggled in school and it kept getting worse and worse," she answered. "Then I failed almost all of my semester exams after first semester of my sophomore year. My friends who were on medication told me I should consider taking meds for attention. I went home and told my other what my friends had said. She answered that I have cousins on both sides who were ADHD and I probably was, too," she said.

"So, you got on medication. How did you know that it was working?" I inquired.

"The best indicator was my final exam grades at the end of the year. I made four "A's" and two "B's". It was so different. I could actually learn things easier."

"Could you tell any other differences?"

"Sometimes when I forgot to take on of my pills, my friends would ask if I forgot. They said I didn't seem to listen to them or that I seemed spacey," she answered.

Alena

Alena, a high school senior, came to me for testing in order to get accommodations for taking tests. She had already been diagnosed with ADHD. I asked her to tell me in her own words what she felt before she was prescribed medication, and how she felt after starting ADHD medication. This is what she said in her own words:

I remember always being frustrated with doing work. Everything felt impossible. I would think I knew how to do it, but it was wrong because I was only grasping half of the concept instead of all of it. My attention span was never long enough for a whole lesson, because I blocked it out. I would be in class and I noticed I just wasn't hearing what was being said. If I tried really hard, I could still hear nothing; I don't know how that worked, but it did. For a long time, a teacher would give directions, but I still wouldn't understand how to do it. I would need a straightforward list step by step of what I needed to do. The more information given to explain something, the more confused I got, but for the other kids it would make more sense. Something big that I still struggle with is reading. That's the only thing that hasn't really gotten easier with medicine. With my medicine, I can focus and get fully into my work and complete it. While other kids could read out loud in class and explain what it meant, I forgot everything I read while reading it. Nothing stuck. I still notice it takes me much longer to finish a passage for class because of my struggle with understanding of what the passage is saying. Even with readings about topics I was interested in, I couldn't remember a single sentence. When I take my medicine, however, I remember things much easier—still not perfect, but improvement nonetheless.

I also have noticed in my math class throughout the years, with all the steps, I find myself lost— not able to find where I left off and then having an entire paper full of work for a simple question. I don't know why I do this, and I think in turn, it just confuses me. I'm much happier now, because of my medicine, I'm able to understand and grasp concepts in and out of school. Understanding concepts makes a world of difference in things you might not have even thought of. I was embarrassed to ask questions when it was "easy" for everyone else. It made me feel alone and frustrated; it added more stress to my life and made me feel stupid. Sometimes, I didn't think I deserved to understand it, since I was the only one who was confused.

Today, I feel much better about my focusing and comprehension related struggles, thanks to many tutors, practice, and medicine. What I'm able to accomplish today, I couldn't even begin working on back then before medication. I needed guiding so I could get from point A to point B, but now by myself, I'm able to make all the connections and exceed them.

Overfocused ADHD

Students who are inattentive but have difficulty shifting their focus of attention fall into this category. These students often have negative thoughts about themselves and tend to worry a great deal. Others may tell them that they worry too much about things. Sometimes, they can be argumentative, especially with their parents. They tend to be inflexible. Some students may have some hyperactivity, but others may not. These students may hold grudges and don't see options in situations. They are opinionated and might not listen to others' opinions or ideas. They frequently need to have things done a certain way or they become upset.

John

John was struggling in college. He was very bright, but it seemed that he just couldn't get it all together. He knew he was intelligent, yet he couldn't pass his classes sometimes just because he couldn't seem to turn in any of the assignments for the class. After he missed one or two assignments, he felt that he couldn't pass the class so "Why try?" When he attended class, he could understand what was being taught, but frequently he couldn't get out of bed in time to get to class. Even though he told himself at the beginning of the semester that he was going to change and he wasn't going to miss any classes, he just couldn't follow through. His parents didn't know what to do. They moved him home and enrolled him in a local community college, where he seemed to be interested in his classes. They hired a tutor who helped him with whatever he needed and helped him stay on track with his classes. He reported that he was doing better, and they had high hopes that this setting was going to work.

Then at the end of the semester, he let them know that he was failing anyway and was going to go into the military. They were disappointed but felt that nothing else was working anyway. They were worried about his entering the military because of the possibility of active duty in a dangerous country, but they did not say anything. They were supportive of his decision. On the night before he was to report, he decided he couldn't go. So, he didn't. Instead, he said he was going to get a job and try to do something with his life. They were also supportive of that decision. Besides, what were they going to do? His parents felt that John was possibly ADHD and in need of medication, but they tried that and it was unsuccessful. I suggested that they schedule an appointment with a professional who specializes in ADHD medication. Even John was on board with the suggestion. After a couple of months, John was prescribed the *correct* medication for his difficulty, and it made a significant change in his life. He was able to follow through on plans, and even enrolled in a night course, where he easily completed all of the assignments. He studied for tests and ended up passing the course with a "B" average. He even amazed himself. He told a friend that he actually *wanted* to go to class and to study. Before medication, he procrastinated with everything to the point of not doing assignments and not attending class. If John had gotten the right help that he needed earlier, he probably would have completed his degree.

Natalie

Natalie was a freshman when I started working with her. When we worked on her math homework, I never really noticed any issues with focus nor attention. She was engaged in all of the problems we had to do. She was organized and always knew exactly what we needed to work on each session.

Then Natalie started having difficulty finishing tests at school. If she did finish, she didn't have time to go back over her work to check. She worked hard. She studied hard.

Natalie took the PSAT in October of her junior year. She didn't do as well as she wanted---what student does? She rationalized that it was very difficult and she ran out of time. I discussed the possibility of testing to determine if she had a processing speed difficulty.

She took her first ACT in December of 2018. She almost didn't tell me her scores, because she felt that they were so low. As it turns out, her scores were on the low end of the average range, but her expectation for herself was always considerably higher. She ran out of time on all of the sections. It was then that she asked her mother to be tested again. She had been tested many years earlier.

When the testing was complete, it definitely indicated that she had a processing speed difficulty. She will request extended time on the ACT. If she is awarded extended time from the ACT committee, it will make a huge difference on the next ACT. The test will be a more accurate assessment of her true abilities.

Natalie may be an excellent candidate for medication. Because medication helps with focus and attention, it generally helps with processing speed. If a student does not have to read and then reread, he can move faster.

Processing speed is directly related to attention and focus difficulties. According to Dr. Clifford Corman, M.D. and Dr. Lawrence Greenberg, M.D. (<u>All You Ever Wanted to Know About Attention Deficits but Didn't Know Whom to Ask...</u>), ADHD is "actually a neurological condition in which the brain (more specifically the frontal lobe) processes information too slowly and inconsistently." It is for this reason that processing speed is an important area to analyze. Slow processing speed can affect all areas in the academic environment.

Nathan

Nathan was the most negative student that I had ever worked with. His mother told me that they were used to his negativity. She said that if Nathan doesn't get his way, he gets very angry. She gives in most of the time to avoid an explosion. Any time she asks Nathan to do something, no matter how simple, he refuses to do it.

I explained to her in a private conversation that most children actually do what their parent asks of them the first time without a fight. Not all, but most. Nathan also had difficulty shifting his attention from one activity to another. If he started working on a project that was due in a week, he would work on it until 2:00 am letting all of his other homework go. Then he didn't have time to do his homework, so he didn't do it. He couldn't schedule his time to fit his homework and projects. His mother would try to talk to him about that, but he wouldn't even listen. He had his own opinion and he wouldn't change.

His mother had no idea that Nathan's negativity and argumentative behavior was actually a type of ADHD. She had no idea that his behavior could be changed with the right medication and supplements. Nathan didn't respond well to medication so his doctor suggested a routine of St. John's Wort to increase his natural serotonin level. Later, another mild medication was added that seemed to work well. Nathan's parents noticed a significant change in his behaviors including his negativity.

Temporal Lobe ADHD

The Temporal Lobe ADHD student has both memory and learning problems. Frequently they have auditory processing difficulties. These students can be irritable with quick bursts of temper. Sometimes the temper tantrums explode into a rage before subsiding. Sometimes there are panic attacks or fear. There may be signs of spaciness or confusion. Students with this diagnosis may have visual changes where they see objects changing shapes or shadows. They may exhibit mild paranoia or sensitivity. Often, they experience headaches or stomach aches for no apparent reason. Some cases indicate a previous head injury. Another characteristic of temporal lobe ADHD may include homicidal or suicidal thoughts.

John

One of the parents with whom I worked told me the situation concerning her son. He struggled all the way through school. His parents tried various medications, but some of them made him feel bad, and he quit taking them. He was irritable, had mood swings, and his temper was on a short fuse. His parents sometimes walked on egg shells around him, so they wouldn't set his anger off. He struggled with learning disabilities. Then one day, their doctor found the right medication and their son flourished. He was in college by this time, and he started doing well. In fact, his grades increased to where he was making all A's. After doing so well for a time, he actually thought he didn't need the medication any longer. He took himself off the medication only to find out that in a couple of months he was back to failing tests and not getting work completed. He went back on the medication and his grades started going up again. One would think this would be a pattern that he could figure out, but he didn't. After doing well again, he decided he had outgrown his need for ADHD medication, so he stopped taking it again. His grades started going downhill once again. With help from his parents, he realized that his ADHD situation was never going to change and while he attended college classes, he would need to continue with medication. Once he graduates, he will need to determine if he can continue in a profession without medication, or if he will be one of the adults who actually needs to continue indefinitely.

Allen

Allen was a student in high school when he started having enough difficulty with school that he didn't want to go. If he even got out of bed, he would arrive at school but would stay in his car instead of going inside. Later, we found out that he was being bullied and the interaction was more than he could handle. The teachers and administrators bent over backward trying to get him to attend school and tried several things to help him catch up with his school work. They made it appear like a reasonable task to him, so that he would try and wouldn't just give up entirely. They even reduced the amount of make-up work that was required. Just when the school professionals and the parents thought everything was going to work out, it didn't. The parents were totally devastated. Allen was their only child.

In working with the parents, we decided that Allen suffered from ADHD and specifically from Temporal Lobe ADHD. Before getting help, Allen had learning problems, showed irritability, had periods of quick temper with little provocation and often misinterpreted comments as negative, when they were not. There were instances when his irritability built and then he would explode. He exhibited many physical symptoms such as headaches and stomach aches that became his excuse to stay at home. Unfortunately, he also had suicidal thoughts. My heart goes out to any student who suffers so much that these symptoms manifest.

Fortunately, the parents were able to enroll Allen in a boarding school near the Austin area that specifically addressed the needs of troubled students. The school provided extensive counseling services and a buddy or a "big-brother" system. The school had several horses and the students learned to care for them. The students grew many of their own vegetables and learned to cook for the others. The education element was provided by computer programming on an individual basis. This environment was perfect for Allen. He was able to return to his parents' home and enroll in a small private school after one year of being at the ranch. The small, private school environment was perfect for him and he was very successful. He struggled to compete his assignments because of his ADHD, but he eventually competed everything and graduated. With a high school diploma under his belt, he decided not to attend college classes. Instead, he chose to go into a business where he is quite successful and is feeling quite good. He continues taking ADHD medication every day. He said he can really tell the difference in his motivation level. He said he wants to do well in his job and feels good about himself now.

Limbic ADHD

Students who fall into this category appear to have a low-grade of sadness or negativity. They may appear more socially isolated or have feelings of hopelessness or worthlessness. They show chronic low self-esteem They may exhibit low energy. These students are no longer interested in things that they were interested in before. Many times, they have difficulty with changes in sleep patterns. They either sleep too much or too little. Dr. Amen states that this category is where ADD and depression intersect each other. He adds that "Limbic ADD is often responsible for failed marriages. The low sexual interest, tiredness, feelings of being constantly overwhelmed, and lack of attention to detail often cause marital conflict. Treating Limbic ADD can literally save families and change a person's life."

Deborah

Deborah was a high school student whose parents drove over 300 miles to have me evaluate her. She was fifteen years old and did pretty well in school. Her grades were in the high B and low A range in every subject. The normal, causal conversation I engage in to help the student feel more relaxed didn't seem to have an effect on Deborah. She didn't appear nervous or anxious; she just didn't have any reaction at all. She never had any facial expressions. Attempts to get her to engage in a conversation went nowhere. She answered the questions I asked but offered no further information. I expected some level of autism. Her test results didn't indicate any level of learning disability or learning difference. Mild indicators were present for inattention. In the test results conference with her parents, I found out that Deborah was always extremely moody and was negative about everything in her life. Her parents didn't enjoy being around her because of her moodiness and negativity. Attempts to have her see a counselor were unsuccessful.

Deborah did not have friends who came over to visit, and she never went to anyone else's house to visit. She was not invited to parties but never seemed to care. She didn't have an interest in cultivating friends and seemed to be content with staying at home in her bedroom. She didn't have any hobbies and wasn't interested in anything that her parents tried to get her interested in.

Her parents thought she might be depressed, so they took her to her doctor for possible medication. A significant trial with medication didn't seem to improve anything.

Deborah lacked motivation. She studied enough to make good grades but was not motivated to have a straight A report card. When her parents talked to her about doing some small jobs to make extra money, she wasn't interested. She had no drive, and they worried that she might spend the rest of her life with no motivation to do anything productive. She just didn't seem to care.

I felt that since medication for depression wasn't successful, and because many of the characteristics of Limbic ADHD were prevalent, I decided that Deborah should consult with her physician for ADHD medication to address Limbic ADHD difficulties. Amino acid supplements have also helped many people with Limbic ADHD.

After Deborah had been on supplements that included amino acids, she gradually started improving. Her negativity appeared to decrease, and she slowly became more social. She seems to be on a slow but steady incline to a more positive and social outlook. Her parents reported that she seems to care more about her grades and doing better in school for the first time ever.

Dr. Amen, M.D. often places patients on DL-phenylalanine and L-tyrosine which are amino acid building blocks for norepinephrine and dopamine---the main two neurotransmitters implicated in this type of ADHD.

Ring of Fire ADHD

Students who are inattentive and easily distracted along with being irritable and overly sensitive may fall into this category. These students are often sensitive to noise, clothes, touch, or light. These students tend to be moody and oppositional. They may show signs of hyperactivity, but they may not. Some of them are inflexible in their thinking and demand to have their way even when told "no" multiple times. They show irritability. There can be periods of mean, nasty or insensitive behavior. Talkativeness and increased impulsivity are often noticed. Sometimes, these students have grandiose ideas. They are unpredictable and may talk fast. Sometimes, they may appear anxious and fearful.

Jeremy

Jeremy was a young student who came in for testing when his teachers referred him for classroom difficulties.

In the parent conference, it was explained that Jeremy had to sleep with a certain blanket that was extremely soft. He couldn't wear certain shirts and sweaters, because they felt scratchy. He couldn't tolerate tags in his clothing. He couldn't wear jeans, if they weren't soft enough. His mother never knew what to buy him to wear, and it became increasingly more frustrating.

He was extremely sensitive to noise. He couldn't go to the movie theater, because the sound was too loud. He often covered his ears to block out sounds. In school, any sounds coming from the hallway interrupted him totally.

Blake Taylor wrote a book titled, <u>ADHD and Me</u>, about what it was like growing up with ADHD issues. He writes about noise sensitivities: "The loud, sharp noises hurt my ears, unlike any other child's in the classroom. They are like needles piercing my eardrums, and they keep me from concentrating or thinking clearly." This explains how some students with Ring of Fire ADHD have sensitivities with loud sounds.

In addition, Jeremy exhibited the normal ADHD symptoms. With help from his pediatrician, Jeremy was placed on ADHD medication and his symptoms subsided over time. He was able to focus easier, and he wasn't as distracted. His sensitivity with clothing also subsided.

Meredith

Meredith was a young child when I tested her. Her mother explained that Meredith was extremely sensitive to sounds. When they went to the movie theatre, Meredith covered her ears because the sound was always too loud. They quit going. She was also very sensitive to her clothing. She had difficulty wearing socks, because she could feel the seams. Any labels on the inside of her shirts had to be removed. She could only wear cotton pajamas and only if they were very soft. She wore the same t-shirt to bed for several years, because it was the only one soft enough. Meredith talked continuously. She tended to be argumentative. Sometimes she could be mean to her little brother and sister. They got on her nerves, and she became irritable. Her mother said that the family walked on egg shells around her, because they didn't want to "set her off."

In addition to behavior difficulties, Meredith struggled at school. She was inattentive and missed out on much of the instruction. She was disorganized and never knew where anything was. She failed to turn in homework and much of the time didn't know what the assignment was. All of the testing and the parent interview pointed to ADHD difficulties. Meredith's mother consulted with the physician who prescribed medication. The medication had to be tweaked until the right dosage was determined, but it worked. Meredith seemed to settle down and didn't pick fights with her siblings. She started making better grades in school and seemed to have more friends.

Anxious ADHD

In addition to the usual inattention, distraction, and disorganization, students in this category tend to be very anxious and tense. They always predict the worst for themselves. These students can get very anxious with timed tests and actually have a panic attack during the test. These students have social anxiety and don't know how to act around other groups of people. Sometimes, they may freeze in social situations. They hate speaking in public and they get very nervous if they have to do so. Many times, these students have physical problems such as headaches or stomach aches. They are very conflict avoidant. They fear being judged. Hyperactivity may or may not be present with students in this category.

Rich

I started tutoring this student after I tested him. I advised the parents to schedule an appointment with a medical doctor who is very knowledgeable in the area of ADHD. Meanwhile, I tutored Rich for the SAT. When he first came, I asked him whether or not he was going to also take the ACT. After forty years of tutoring for both tests, I have come to the conclusion that the ACT is often the better test for many students. He replied that he couldn't take the ACT, because he had already spent so much time preparing for the SAT, and that it would be time wasted. "No," I answered. "When you study for one, you are studying for both. Your time will not have been wasted at all. The only difference is the format of the test. You still need your brain and all that knowledge for both tests! I suggest you take both tests and see which one you like better!"

Another reason Rich was pulling away from taking the ACT was that he was awarded extended time to take the SAT, but accommodations weren't requested for the ACT.

So, what does Rich's ADHD look like? He is extremely disorganized. Papers are in disarray on his work area. Things fall to the floor and are left there. He reminds me of the character Pigpen in the Peanuts comics. When he takes notes, his notes are very sloppy. Actually, he doesn't know how to take notes. When he leaves, I know those notes are going to go into a black hole somewhere, so I decided to keep his notes in my office until the time for him to study for the test. He does not come in with any of the paperwork I handed him the first session. I don't even know if he knows where it is now.

He also makes numerous appointments and then forgets about them. When I remind him through text message to his mother, he invariably changes the time or the day. He also makes double appointments on the same day and the same time with other tutors. His mother does what she can to keep him on track, but even *she* cannot keep him straight!

Rich is in constant motion. His leg is moving so much while he is taking practice problems that his whole workbook is moving. He doesn't seem to notice. He told me that he doesn't get enough sleep. I know he is getting good nutrition, because his mother is adamant about that, but his sleep is lacking. I've explained how important sleep is for his brain, but he doesn't seem to change anything.

I've never seen a student so driven. It's good to be driven, but I worry about the intense pressure he may be putting on himself. He always talks about failure and not doing well. He has many worries. He has said many times, "I'm afraid I'm not going to do well on the test." He always predicts the worse. "You don't think I can do well, do you?" he asks me.

Rich also has many physical problems that are symptoms of stress. He has had to discontinue tests before because of panic attacks. He sometimes has headaches, stomach aches, and gastrointestinal issues.

Although he has improved significantly, he still tends to have difficulties in social situations. He would like to have a girlfriend but doesn't have the social skills to make it happen. Earlier in his life, he was unable to talk to other students or be involved in any social situation. He has come a long way.

Rich is the typical classic ADHD student but when Dr. Amen added a seventh type of ADHD to his latest book, it seemed to fit Rich perfectly. The list of symptoms includes the core ADD symptoms plus: frequently anxious or nervous, physical stress symptoms such as headaches, tends to freeze in social situations, dislikes or gets excessively nervous speaking in public, predicts the worse, conflict avoidant, and fear of being judged.

His parents confirmed that he has all of the aforementioned symptoms. I saw many of them myself in the tutoring sessions.

Although he shows to have most of these symptoms, there may be more than ADHD going on here. There may be some depression and other factors. I depend on the medical doctor to help solve the puzzle. Rich says that the ADHD medicine is helping him considerably. He went from making mostly "B's" in school to making straight "A's." He even received a letter at the end of the school year commending him for making the top 10% of the student population for grade point average.

By tutoring him, I realized he also had gaps in his learning. He was able to do some very difficult math problems but also missed problems he should have learned how to do in eighth grade. I can only surmise, like with so many other

ADHD students, that his inattention caused him to miss out on learning.

Cannon

Cannon is my great-nephew. Since he was having difficulty in his school setting and appeared to falling further and further behind his classmates, his mother asked for him to be tested for learning disabilities.

I conducted the usual psychoeducational evaluation which indicated several learning disabilities along with significant attention and processing speed difficulties. I went to the doctor along with Cannon and his mother to see what the pediatrician would prescribe. His doctor looked through the report and then said his "go to" medication for ADHD was Concerta. He always started his students on a low dosage and then monitored then closely every two weeks until the dosage appeared to be adequate to handle the difficulty. Cannon showed immediate results. His teachers noticed a significant improvement. His mother reported improved behaviors. However, he still appeared tired most of the time and he had dark circles under his eyes.

Two years went by and then Cannon had a visit with his dentist to consider braces. It was determined that his mouth was too small and his teeth did not have the necessary room. Then it was discovered that his trachea was so small that he was not getting enough oxygen at night while sleeping. A sleep test at the sleep clinic indicated a significant blockage and frequent sleep interruptions throughout the night. His mother was told that Cannon's ADHD might not be ADHD at all but sleep and oxygen deprivation throughout the night. He was put on a sleep machine (CPAP) and his appearance started improving. He felt better and his dark circles under his eyes diminished.

According to the doctor, Cannon will need surgery to rebuild his jaw, throat and trachea. Evidently, this problem was never detected when his physician looked in his mouth or his throat during exams. In the meantime, the sleep machine is helping significantly and he feels better.

Then things changed again. He started challenging his mother on everything. He became disrespectful and talked back to her often. When she tried to discipline him, he screamed and yelled at her. She received texts from school telling her how disruptive he was on those particular days. He was punished at school, but it didn't seem to help. His mother was at wits end. When I suggested that she consult her physician for a stronger ADHD medication, she was hesitant. She didn't want to put her son on medication in the first place and now it looked like he needed something stronger. Her physician decided on Adderall. She hated the idea of putting her son on Adderall. I finally convinced her to give it a try. After all, they couldn't continue like this, could they? The stronger medication did help and the defiance subsided.

It may be that he needs both the sleep machine and also the medication to fully function in his educational setting.

David-not ADHD

My great-nephew's case reminded me of a test case I had several years ago. A high school student was referred to me, because he couldn't focus. He made good grades and was never a disruption, but had trouble focusing on homework, and it always took forever to complete. In talking with him, he told me that he fell asleep in every class at school. I thought maybe he was exaggerating, so I asked if he fell asleep after lunch. He explained that he fell asleep in EVERY class.

"What do your teachers think of that?" I asked him.

"I don't think they really care, because I make good grades," he responded.

I couldn't believe that the message didn't get around among his teachers and something wasn't said to his parents. Maybe the teachers didn't want everyone to know that he slept in their classrooms.

As I was testing him, I reached down to pick up a test from the bottom drawer of my desk. When I straightened up, I could clearly see that he was asleep. I very quietly sat there to determine how long it would take him to wake up. In a very short time, he acted startled and woke himself up. I reported the incident to his mother. This was clearly not normal. I told her about his sleeping in every class. She took him to a sleep center and it was determined that he had a severe sleep disorder—sleep apnea—and would require intervention with a CPAP machine. She later reported that he was doing well, and that they were looking at other options, since he would be going off to college in the fall. I know sleep apnea can be deadly, and I was relieved that his parents were on top of the situation.

Robert

Robert was a student who was a senior at a prestigious private high school. He was very motivated and very driven, but no matter how hard he studied, couldn't make the grades he wanted. He seemed to always run out of time and had to rush through the end of tests to get finished. When I tested him, I found that he was an over-achiever. The testing showed that he had a significant processing speed problem and that he would qualify for extended time. In addition, he showed all the characteristics of ADHD-Inattention. I recommended he be evaluated for medication through a physician who could also address his issues of depression. With medication and in less than two months, Robert's grades improved to all "A's" and he seemed happier. He received a letter from his school at the end of the year saying he was on the special honor roll for high grades.

Many, many times when I test a student and find that he or she is struggling with ADHD difficulties, I learn that one of the parents has the same issue. Many times, the parent wasn't diagnosed because when he or she was a child, diagnosis was more difficult or nonexistent. Now, we are learning more and more about attention and focus difficulties and diagnosis is much more prevalent. When I encounter parents who have difficulty finishing the questionnaires and the paperwork requested when testing their child, I suspect ADHD might be the culprit. Since ADHD runs in families, that is another aspect to consider.

William

William came to me for tutoring for ACT/SAT preparation. He was a delightful student and very mannerly. In a short period of time, I could tell that William was ADHD. In a conversation with his mother, she confirmed that he had been diagnosed with ADHD earlier and had been on medication for some time but was not currently taking medication. When I asked him about it, he said that he didn't know exactly why he stopped taking it, because he remembered it helped him. Sometimes parents will discontinue medication if they are not seeing an increase in grades, or if they do not think it is working for the student. I asked William if he could begin retaking his medication and that I thought it could make a significant difference. I discussed it with his mother. He took medication the last couple of months of his junior year and said it made a significant difference. He said, "I can't really explain it, but I learn so much more. I listen in class, and I don't talk to my friends as often. It's hard to explain, but it makes me learn." When a student can tell a difference that is this significant, he really needs to stay on medication throughout his academic career.

Mary Ann

Mary Ann was a student I worked with for several years. When I first started with her, I could tell she had some severe focus and attention difficulties. I asked if she had ever been diagnosed with ADHD. She said she was dyslexic and also ADHD. She said she no longer took medication, because some of her friends said she was mean when she took her medication. If a medication is right for a student, the side effects should be minimal or nonexistent. It should be more seamless. It's often difficult to find the right medication, so it is important to have a physician who knows how to prescribe or adjust prescriptions to fit the individual. I encouraged her parents to try to find the right medication for her, because her academics were suffering from her focus and inattention difficulties. When that step was finally taken and done so successfully, Mary Ann became a different student. Her grades went up and her friends did not complain about her personality.

ADHD is usually more prevalent while a student is in an academic setting. When the student is asked to turn in papers on time, study for tests, complete assignments, the ADHD student struggles. There are many professions, once the student is out of school, where ADHD is not as noticeable. Any profession without strict timelines seems to work better for ADHD adults. Or, any profession where another individual such as a secretary, assistant, or bookkeeper handles the paperwork or keeps the ADHD adult on the right schedule seems to work well. Someone else needs to have the responsibility for the organization and schedule.

Chapter Five
Adult ADHD Diagnosis

ADHD in adults is usually easy to diagnose. Although there is variation in characteristics of many adults with ADHD, adults with ADHD usually have great difficulty in getting anywhere on time. Their brains do not have the internal brain clock that is common in other people. They cannot plan ahead in order to figure out when they must leave in order to arrive on time. They can get distracted wherever they are, which causes them to leave late, which then causes them to be late to their appointment. No amount of cajoling or reprimanding or screaming will make them understand how it disturbs others. Usually other people give up, too. They either take another car or avoid confrontation entirely.

ADHD adults usually live in a very cluttered environment. Stacks of papers and books or files get higher and higher

116

on the kitchen table or in the corner of the dining room. They can never get around to going through the stacks to throw out unwanted items. The clutter gets worse and worse. Even the refrigerator and freezer become packed with more and more items, many of which should be thrown out or are no longer edible.

Sometimes closet or cabinet doors cannot be closed, because there is so much in the closet preventing the closure. Garages cannot be used to house vehicles, because they are full of clutter.

Often adults with ADHD have at least one paid storage unit. They may have two or three as their belongings multiply. They cannot make the decision of letting things go. Instead, they just keep piling them up. I have known many people who have paid far more in storage unit rent than what the entire contents were worth. In other cases, the person pays the rent for years, only to finally get rid of everything in the unit at some point.

In houses or offices of adults with ADHD, there are usually no surfaces that are free of clutter. They don't want anyone else to clean the surfaces, because they want to "go through" the stuff first. Then, of course, they never do.

Adult ADHD individuals usually stay "on the go." They leave their home, because if they stay there, they would be expected to clear at least some of the clutter. They don't know HOW to get started. They don't know WHERE to get started. If they leave, they don't have to think about it. As one adult ADHD person told me, "It's easier to drive away from it than working on it and getting frustrated."

Adults with ADHD usually have great difficulty finishing projects. They get too distracted to complete anything. They will *start* many projects, however.

Adults with ADHD tend to talk excessively. It is not uncommon that the person on the other end of the phone line is not talking at all. In fact, it may be difficult to get one word into the conversation. One time, I decided to stay on the line with an ADHD friend to determine just how long he would continue talking. Since that would actually drive me crazy, I walked around the house doing some of the work I needed to do. I said nothing more than "uh huh…yes…uh huh." I was on the phone for more than two hours straight.

I witnessed my husband actually fall asleep while talking to his sister. She talked constantly without any reaction from him, until he actually fell asleep with the phone propped up. The phone was propped up to his ear, but he was sound asleep. That one-sided conversation continued for quite some time.

One of the most amazing things about ADHD adults is their tendency to argue. I would have never believed that this was a legitimate characteristic had I not seen it in Dr. Daniel Aman's book titled, <u>Healing ADD: The Breakthrough Program That</u>

Allows You to See and Heal the 7 Types of ADD.

I have seen this in real life. The ADHD person keeps egging on his unwilling suspect, until that person actually starts screaming at him. The screaming actually stimulates the ADHD person and he gets satisfaction from that. Really? That doesn't even make sense BUT IT IS TRUE! I've witnessed it many, many times in my own family!

I have to quote Dr. Amen, M.D. on this one. In Chapter Fourteen: The Games ADD People Play is a section called "I Bet I Can Get You to Yell At Me or Hit Me." I'm not joking.

According to Dr. Amen, M.D., "Many people with ADD are masterful at getting others to scream, yell, spank, and basically fly out of control. They get others so upset that they cannot help but lose it. These negative behaviors provide quite an adrenaline rush but frequently lead to serious negative consequences, such a divorce, fights at school, unemployment, and even abuse. Again, the game is unconscious, not planned. It seems as if the ADD person senses the most vulnerable issues for others, and they work on them until there is an explosion." (p. 180).

I saw this vividly in my own family. The telephone rings. My husband answers. Within a few minutes, I hear him scream and yell at his sister. He completely loses his patience. He finally hangs up. His brother does the same thing with the same family member--- their sister. When I read them the section of Dr. Amen's book cited above, they couldn't believe it. From that point forward, they tried to remain calm when talking to their sister on the phone. Even though she had a way of inciting the same intense anger, they worked very, very hard to control the anger on their end. They tried to talk in a normal voice and not scream at her. Most of the time it didn't work. She was a lot better at that game than they were at avoiding it.

Dr. Amen addresses that phenomenon by saying that if the spouse or sibling can remain nonreactive for a long enough period of time, the conflict-driven behavior usually significantly diminishes.

In addition, ADHD in adults include frequent job changes, difficulty managing a checkbook, depression over underachievement, and also frequent changes and moves.

For those adults who are considered senior citizens, ADHD is usually not diagnosed. Other people consider the symptoms to be a sign of dementia or personality problems. But, when these older adults isolate themselves or have problems with their health because they forget to take their medication, it might be ADHD instead of dementia. It is difficult to tell.

Dr. Harvey Davisson, Ph.D. provides the following list of symptoms for adult ADD/ADHD:

Disorganization

Lack of focus

Losing things

Social conflicts

Impulsiveness

Low self-esteem

Frustration

Sleep disorders

Mood swings

Defensiveness

Anxiety

Hyperactivity

Addictive behavior

Have someone in the family with ADD, manic-depressive illness, depression, or other disorders

Dr. Davisson, Ph.D. is the director of the ADD/ADHD Center and the Davisson Clinic.

Chapter Six
Adult ADHD Stories

Although most students will drop off medication once they graduate from an academic setting, there are a few people who remain on medication as adults. Sometimes, they have never been on medication. I have several interesting stories to tell about some of the adults with whom I have had the pleasure of working.

Dr. Mary Jones

One adult was Dr. Mary Jones. I got a call from Dr. Jones on a Thursday afternoon. She explained that she was a D.O. physician and had to be evaluated every seven years by the licensing board. She had to have extended time in order to take the tests, but she needed documentation in the form of a complete psychoeducation evaluation in order to get extended time on the tests. In order to keep her license, she had to take the test by the following month. Since the licensing agency took approximately one month to approve the request and review the psychoeducational evaluation, she needed to be tested immediately. She wondered if I could do the testing the *next day*.

There is no professional in the Dallas area who can usually do testing the very next day and then do the grading, analysis, and report writing to have it ready in order to fax to the Board on Monday!! If it couldn't be done, Dr. Jones would miss her licensing test, and she would not be able to see patients for several months.

That meant I would have to do the testing on Friday, stay up until late grading and analyzing the results, and then start typing the report. I would have to compete the report by Sunday evening. In addition, I had other students to tutor on both Saturday and Sunday, but I agreed to test her. "Can you get here at 8:00 in the morning?" I asked her. She came.

Knowing that processing speed was an issue for her and knowing that processing speed goes hand-in-hand with ADHD, I asked her if she had ever been diagnosed. She told me she had not. Based on the fact that she waited until the very last minute to get her testing done when her license was at stake was a red flag. That is what ADHD people do!

At some point in the time we had together, Dr. Jones explained that she had taken Organic Chemistry at least six times. I made a mental note of that.

As the testing progressed, I kept identifying characteristics that are typical of ADHD individuals. I waited to say anything until after I had completed the testing and had time to look at the results as a whole.

On Sunday evening when I had finally finished the complete evaluation, I called her on the phone to go over the test results with her. I usually go over the test results in person, but she lived over 50 miles away, so it was more convenient over the phone.

I told her, "Everything is pointing to ADHD difficulties."

It was at that point that she gave out a sigh and said, "You're right. I've known it all along. I guess I just deny it, but it's true. I've had ADD my whole life."

"Have you ever tried medication? If you had, you wouldn't have had to take Organic Chemistry six times." I mentioned.

"No," she said. "I've never tried medication. But I do know that in every job that I've been in, they have always given me the best secretary who knows how to manage my issues. My secretary keeps me on track. When I worked for myself, I lost so much money, because I saw a lot of patients but would never bill them. I could never get organized enough to bill patients. I really think I am a good doctor, and I know I help my patients, but

I just have to realize that someone else has to do everything for me as far as the business part is concerned."

I realize that Dr. Jones could have had a much easier time while in college if she had just had some help with her ADHD difficulty. She only became a doctor, because she was *so* motivated and *so* determined. Even so, it took her several years longer to get through medical school. Something as simple as medication could have made her life so much easier—and she is a medical doctor!

Louise

Louise was the mother of one of my students. I tested her son. His test results showed obvious ADHD difficulties, so I recommended a medical doctor to help with medication. She didn't tell me until later that when she went to the doctor with her son, everything that the doctor said about her son's problem actually applied to her as well. She listened carefully. Then, once medication was prescribed, Louise took one of her son's pills.

When she told me, she said, "I know it is illegal and I know I shouldn't have done it, but I just had to see if it would do anything for me. Since my son and I are about the same height and weight, I figured it would be OK."

"Well," I said. "What happened?"

"I thought it would take several days, but I noticed a change right away." Then sweeping her hand across her forehead, she said, "It was like someone just cleared all of the cobwebs out of my head. I could think so clearly and it was obvious."

Since she noticed a significant difference, she decided to go back to the doctor to get medication for herself.

Joan

Joan was another mother who learned that she had ADHD by attending the doctor's visit with her son.

She told me this story: "Growing up, I was always very smart. I had to work hard, but I learned things pretty quickly. I did well enough in school to get a full ride scholarship to a nice university. I never went. I procrastinated enough that the scholarship was rescinded. When I married, I always had trouble keeping house. I had clutter everywhere. My excuse was that I was taking care of a husband and three children. I could never get anywhere on time. I was late everywhere I went. Eventually, we always took separate cars to church or anywhere really, because my family didn't want to be late all the time.

I never really understood why they were so irritated with me. But they were. Then when the kids went to school, I tried to hold down a job. I could never stay in a job very long—getting fired for being late or not being organized or not being able to complete projects. I finally gave up trying to get another job. I also went through a divorce at the request of my husband.

It wasn't until I attended that doctor's appointment with my son, that I heard various characteristics that also fit me perfectly. I made another appointment and was prescribed medication.

The medication has made a huge difference in my life. Now, I can actually understand WHY my family was frequently irritated with me. I truly believe that I would have never gotten a divorce, if I had only known what was happening to me. But without the medication, I could not reason—I could not understand how others felt.

Now I'm thinking if I had been diagnosed earlier, I probably would have accepted that scholarship to the university. I probably would have been able to keep a job. I would have been a better mother—not angering my family because of my ADHD difficulties. I would have been a better wife, too. In fact, I doubt I would have gotten a divorce if I had been on medication.

All I know now is that if I leave the house in the morning and find myself feeling scattered and not thinking clearly, I realize that I forgot to take my ADHD medication. I turn around and go back home. It is that important."

Mark

Mark was a man in his fifties. He was a professional artist who did very well. He told me that this is what ADHD means for him: "I will decide to walk out to the mail box to get the mail. On the way out, I notice that the plant on the front porch is dying from lack of water. I walk back inside to get a contained to fill with water, so I can water the plants that are dying. I find the container but walking by the utility room reminds me that I have to take the clothes out of the washer to put in the dryer. I finally remember about the plants, so I walk back to the kitchen where I left the watering can. I finally fill it with water to water the plants. I water the plants and go inside to work on my painting. I never remember the mail." He is on medication, or otherwise, he would have those experiences every day. He said that he wouldn't be able to make a living if it weren't for his medication.

Randell

Randell was a dentist who was never officially diagnosed with ADHD. He had many of the symptoms but grew up in the days when ADHD was not well known. When he was in high school, he was late everywhere he went. Even if it meant that he would make others late also, he just couldn't get anywhere on time. His room looked like a crime scene. He finally gave up and just changed the sheets on his bed but didn't even try to organize or clean up his room. He had stacks of stuff everywhere. He played in a band, so his room was filled with equipment of all kinds. Books and music were strewn everywhere. He always claimed that he knew where everything was, as is the case with most ADHD students and adults. Later, when he became a dentist, his office looked pretty much the same. His assistants ventured in at some point and tried to organize his paperwork. His assistants kept him on schedule, but when he was at home and did not have the help of his assistants, he couldn't get anywhere on time. He would tell his friends and family that he was "almost there" when he wouldn't show up for another two hours. He loved to cook, but it took forever. He got distracted and time passed. A 7:00 dinner would be ready at 9:30. It was delicious though! He had trouble sleeping and would frequently stay up until two or three in the morning. Even when he had to work the next day, and had to get up early to get to the office, he had difficulty sleeping.

Doctors aren't sure why people with ADD have more sleep problems than the normal population. Some doctors think it has to do with serotonin, the neurotransmitter most closely tied to Overfocused and Ring of Fire ADD. Everyone depends on serotonin to sleep so when there is not enough serotonin, it makes sleeping very difficult.

Marilyn

Marilyn was the mother of a friend of mine, so I am getting the information through her daughter. When Marilyn was younger, she had tremendous difficulty with being on time. Even when other family members depended on her, she could not get anywhere on time. She was almost fired from her job as a doctor's nursing assistant, because she was late every day. Since the family members shared the family car, someone had to pick her up from work at night. The driver appeared at the time designated only to find that Marilyn would not come out.

The driver waited and waited until finally Marilyn would appear. There was one story where one of her brothers had an important basketball game to play in. Marilyn promised to return with the car since she only needed it for a short time. Her brother waited and waited. He ended up missing the game, and he was one of the most important players. Marilyn's daughter tells how embarrassed she was as an elementary student when her mother couldn't manage to pick up the carpool on time. The children sat on the curb waiting for Marilyn, until someone finally called another parent to pick them up. Of course, that parent was upset and the students were upset. If that only happened once, it would be one thing, but it happened over and over.

As an adult, Marilyn continued her difficulty with timing. On one occasion, she told a friend that she was "one her way" to pick her up. The friend knew Marilyn only lived about six minutes from her house, so she got ready and waited by the door. What the friend didn't know was that Marilyn had not yet taken a shower. She took a shower, got dressed, and appeared at the friend's house over an hour later. She thought nothing of it.

Marilyn's house was always cluttered. She lived in a beautiful home, but most flat surfaces were covered with miscellaneous items. A beautiful sunken tub in the master bath was filled with stacks of magazines and newspapers that she always intended to go through. Once when her adult son tried to help her by eliminating some of the stacks, she became tearful. She just couldn't handle "things" taken from her home. The family downsized. Soon, areas in the new home became so filled with furniture and books and magazincs and stacks that it was difficult to walk through. Her garage was so packed that there was no room for a car or anything else. The moving boxes filled with kitchen items sat in the kitchen for over a year. She had to walk around the box to cook in the kitchen.

Marilyn was one of the most giving individuals in the world. She would "give you the shirt off her back." Really. She always wanted to help others. Once when she volunteered to make the hot sauce for Thanksgiving dinner, she arrived with the freshly made hot sauce when everyone had finished the meal and was eating dessert. "Don't ask her to bring anything! Just try to get her to the meal on time!" Her family learned quickly.

Marilyn's daughter tells of a really funny story that is also very true. Marilyn invited the priest to come to their house for dinner. After dinner, she asked him if he wanted fresh apple pie for dessert. When he smiled at the thought of a fresh piece of homemade apple pie, she nodded and then got in her car to drive to the store to buy the apples. That story has been told a million times. This is not a joke.

One of Marilyn's favorite past times was shopping. Although she had a million things that needed to be done in her home, she almost never stayed there. I mentioned this to another ADHD adult who explained it to me this way: "It is so much easier to leave the house than to stay and face what needs to be done. Leaving means you don't have to make the decision to do something, because you can't make the decision. You don't know where to start. So, leave and you don't have to."

Often ADHD adults have difficulty going to bed at night and they have difficulty getting up in the morning. Marilyn often washed her clothes at two or three in the morning. Because of that, she could not get up the next morning and would sleep until noon. As mentioned earlier, doctors aren't sure why people with ADD have more sleep problems than the normal population. Some doctors think it has to do with serotonin, the neurotransmitter most closely tied to Overfocused and Ring of Fire ADD. Everyone depends on serotonin to sleep so when there is not enough serotonin, it makes sleeping very difficult.

Chapter Seven
My Experience with
Phosphatidylserine

I take many supplements—vitamins, nutrients, and minerals. I trust that some of them are doing the job that they were meant to do. I know some of them are doing their job, because I have negative results if I stop taking them.

After many years playing sports and wearing out my knees, I found that my knees were often painful, and I couldn't kneel down to the floor and then get back up. I could hear my knees pop and crack when I walked up or down stairs. Several times I had what is called a "floater." If you haven't had one of those you don't know what you are missing. A floater is a chip of cartilage that becomes lodged in the knee joint causing extreme pain. When my husband discussed the possibility of having another knee surgery with his orthopedic surgeon, he was told, "If you take glucosamine, you won't need knee surgery." I was there also, so I asked about floaters. His recommendation was to take glucosamine for that, also. My husband and I started taking glucosamine immediately. My husband never had another knee surgery and my knees are fine today—as long as I continue with the supplement. My knees aren't painful, they don't pop and crack on stairs, and I have never had another floater. I am a believer.

I have many more supplements that I rely on daily to maintain my energy level, eye health, etc. I'll need to write another book for that topic. The one supplement that I must tell all readers about is phosphatidylserine.

Since I took supplements for everything else, I asked the salesman in the vitamin store to advise me on supplements for memory and brain health. He took a few minutes to explain why phosphatidylserine would be good for me to take. I bought a bottle and started taking the capsules immediately. I didn't expect any noticeable difference. I didn't think I'd be able to tell an improvement in memory. Then something started happening that was quite surprising.

I was watering the plants in the backyard when I heard a dog bark in the commons area. That bark triggered a memory from over fifty years ago. When I was a young child, I asked my mother if I could have a poodle puppy. She agreed to my request and said that she knew of a lady who raised puppies. The lady's name popped right into my head. I'm terrible with names, so that was a shock to me. Besides, if you are a young child going to pick up a new puppy, do you really pay attention to the lady's name? Since she was not a personal friend of my mother, I probably only heard her name once or twice. That was fifty years ago! The name was Robbie Tharp. Robbie is not a common name for a female, and Tharp is not common. It is usually Thorpe. How did I come up with that name? It could only be the phosphatidylserine. A few days later, someone mentioned the difference between teachers and principals and another name popped into my mind from approximately forty years earlier. Jack Barton was the guy who sat next to me in one of our education classes in school. I never saw him other than in class. When I heard someone mention the difference between teachers and principals, his name popped right into my head. Where did that come from?

In subsequent months, there were numerous times when I was the one who could come up with names of movie stars from the twenties or friends we haven't seen in years and years. My husband would say, "Where did that come from?" or "How did you come up with that?" I'd usually answer, "I'm telling you, it's those pills I'm taking."

Since my mother is twenty years older than I am and has difficulty with memory at times, I bought some phosphatidylserine for her, and she started taking it. Within two weeks, she called to tell me she wasn't taking it any more. She was remembering word-for-word conversations that occurred between her and her mother when she was a young girl. Since those conversations were always very negative, she did not want to relive them again. I tried to explain to my mother that her brain was going through an adjustment period and that she should continue using the pills.

"After a little while, all of that will settle down, and you probably won't relive those conversations. At least we know something is really going on in your brain. I think you should continue," I explained. She would not. She quit taking the pills.

I noticed another thing that the phosphatidylserine helped me with. Every year, my husband and I make Thanksgiving and Christmas dinner for our family. We generally have between 25 and 35 people and we make all of the dishes ourselves. Sometimes, someone brings a dessert, but we prepare to do everything ourselves. It takes several days to set up the extra tables, decorate the tables, set the tables with dishes and silverware, and then cook. Cooking usually starts two days ahead of time. We are exhausted when 6:00pm comes around on the day of the dinner.

After taking phosphatidylserine for some time, I noticed that the dinners weren't as exhausting as they had been for the previous fifteen or so years. I actually had time to rest before the dinner. What was different? We had the same menu every single meal. Sometimes the side dishes would change, but the number was the same. I finally figured out that the phosphatidylserine made me more organized. I was not retracing my steps. I was more efficient. That is the only thing that it could possibly be.

I also started realizing that I could get the very complicated math problems that students brought me when I tutored them. My mathematical skills were enhanced. I could notice the difference.

I also noticed that my memory was so much better in daily activities. When I left my office at the front of my home to go to the other side of the house, I remembered to take what I needed. I didn't find myself having to go back to the office to get what I had forgotten. My brain was simply working more efficiently.

I have been asked if this supplement could be given to children. We decided to research that question. What I found out was that phosphatidylserine is often given to children who have ADHD difficulties when medication is not wanted. There is much research concerning phosphatidylserine that I encourage you to read.

I have been on phosphatidylserine for several years now, and I plan to continue because I know what it has done for me. I know not everyone is the same, so it has to be up to the individual whether he or she takes the supplement or not. I also believe that one bottle won't do the trick. I believe a continual and consistent administration over time is necessary for optimal results.

Chapter Eight
Understanding Medication

Almost every story I wrote about in this book includes medication. Although I am strongly in support of vitamins, nutrients, and minerals, I often encourage trying ADHD medication because of what I have seen over the years of working with students. Some parents are concerned, because they hear that putting a child on medication will promote drug use such as alcohol or marijuana. Actually, the reverse is true. Students who have ADHD who go untreated are usually the ones who turn to drugs and alcohol. One study from Harvard University showed that 52% of untreated ADD adults abuse drugs or alcohol. They often turn to drugs to help with restlessness issues, depression difficulties, anxiety issues, or focus issues. Properly treating students with ADD *now* will actually decrease drug abuse later.

Remember, your physician needs to hear from you concerning side effects and effectiveness of the medication. You have to play an active role.

Summary

Most of the stories in this book tell of students or adults who were identified as ADHD and who overcame their difficulties with the right medication. That is not always the case. I can think of two or three cases where no matter what was tried, nothing seemed to work. In cases like that, it could be that the condition is misdiagnosed as ADD when perhaps it is a thyroid illness. I have always believed that if the right medication were found, and the right dosage were determined, then the end result would be very positive. If the right medication is determined, there should be no side effects or slight side effects after the first week or two. With some medications, lack of appetite may continue. There may be an adjustment time period for some students. Also, even if the right medication is found, there may come a time when it is no longer effective. Students are changing as they grow. Their brains are also changing. It takes a great deal of attention to stay on top of medication needs. It takes the student, the parents, and the medical doctor to ensure the medication is still effective.

One student, Blake Taylor, said that ADHD medicines can help quite a bit. "Without my medicine, I feel aimless, like a tiger in a cage. I have an enormous amount of energy, but I can't focus it and I can't seem to accomplish anything."

If you and your child are suffering because of his difficulties in school, consider ADHD as a possible answer. Don't jump to the conclusion that he is just lazy or isn't trying. Don't jump to the conclusion that he is just disorganized or needs to study more. I've seen too many cases where this just isn't the case. There are simple parent and student questionnaires that can help get you on the right path if ADHD is detected. Look into it!

Also, bright, advantaged students with a strong work ethic may do well in school, although they don't usually work up to their potential. They usually do well, until they encounter more difficult tasks and assignments when they enter high school or college. Some ADHD adults are very productive and very successful in spite of their ADHD.

I encourage you to read any book written by Dr. Daniel Amen, M.D. concerning ADD. He is the expert who utilizes actual brain scans to prove the science behind ADD. A section of his book also addresses natural supplements strategies for ADD types.

I strongly agree with Dr. Amen on several points: The first is that ADHD is a neurological disorder that has strong psychological and social consequences. The second point is that everyone—children, teens, adults, and parents—need to know that it is not their fault. They didn't cause the problem and there is a lot of hope. Finally, family members need to know that they need *good* information and the child, teenager, or adult with ADD needs *good* treatment.

If parents even suspect that there may be an ADHD problem, I strongly encourage you to just check it out. It may turn your life and the life of your child around. If you are an adult, and you suspect *you* may have an ADHD problem, please check it out. It might change your life and the lives of those around you significantly.

I'd also love to hear your personal stories. Please email me at dr.lindasalinas@verizon.net.

References

Amen, Daniel, M.D. *Healing ADD: The Breakthrough Program that Allows You to See and Heal the 7 Types of ADD,* New York: Penguin Random House, 2013.

American Psychiatric Association, *Diagnostic and Statistical Manual of Mental Disorders,* Washington, DC, 2008.

Barkley, R. *Attention-Deficit Hyperactivity Disorder: A Handbook for Diagnosis and Treatment*, second edition, New York: Guilford Press, 1998.

Corman, M.D., Clifford and Lawrence Greenberg, M.D. *All You Ever Wanted to Know about Attention Deficits But Didn't Know Whom to Ask...*California: Universal Attention Disorders, Inc., 1997.

Hallowell, E. and J. Ratey, *Delivered from Distraction,* New York: Ballantine Books, 2005.

Honos-Webb, L. *The Gift of ADHD,* California: New Harbinger Publications, 2005.

Taylor, Blake, *ADHD & Me*, California: New Harbinger Publications, Inc., 2007.

Walker, B. *The Girl's Guide to AD/HD,* Maryland: woodbine Hose, 2005.

Zeigler Dendy, and A. Zeigler, *A Bird's Eye View of Life with ADD and ADHD,* AL: Cherish the Children, 2003.

www.ingramcontent.com/pod-product-compliance
Lightning Source LLC
Chambersburg PA
CBHW061303280526
45784CB00002B/875